Cardiology:
Fast Focus Study Guide

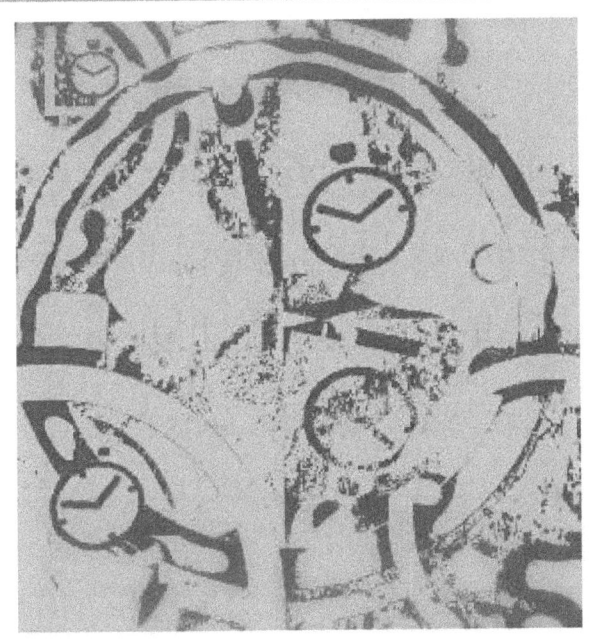

Acknowledgements

I dedicate this book to my beautiful wife and children, who I love more than all the water in all the oceans and all the seas.

CONTENTS

- This book is written for any medical professionals who want to learn more about cardiology.

- There are over 270 pages of easy to read facts about endocrinology.

- The Kindle version of this book was designed to be easily read on your mobile phone. Put the print version of this book in your bathroom or on your coffee table.

- This is the perfect graduation gift for the aspiring physician or graduating physician.

- This Fast Focus Study Guide will provide you with a practical review of the key information you need to know.

- Buy this book now if you want this quick and concise information

In New York Heart Association class I heart failure the patients have no limitations of physical activity.

In New York Heart Association class II heart failure the patients have symptoms with normal activity

In New York Heart Association class III heart failure the patients have symptoms with less than normal activity

In New York Heart Association class IV heart failure the patients have symptoms at rest.

Q waves on EKG are indicative of a transmural infarction.

Infectious endocarditis is the most common cause of aortic insufficiency.

Coronary artery disease is the most common cause of congestive heart failure.

ST depression on EKG is consistent with subendocardial ischemia.

ST elevation on EKG is indicative of transmural ischemia or coronary artery spasm.

T-wave inversion on EKG can be either nonspecific, occur during ischemia, or occur after an MI.

The other name for Mobitz type I is Wenchebach.

Wenchebach is indicated by the presence of progressive lengthening of the PR interval followed by a drop of the QRS.

A Mobitz II is indicated by a constant PR interval with a skip of the QRS

A pacemaker is indicated for Mobitz

type I only if the patient is

symptomatic.

All patients with a Mobitz type II should have a pacemaker placed, even if not symptomatic

Pacemakers should be placed in patients with a symptomatic Mobitz type I, any patient with Mobitz type II, and all patients with a third degree AV block

A first degree AV block is present when there is >.20 second PR interval on the electrocardiogram.

Mitral stenosis is characterized by a diastolic opening snap, loud S1, and a diastolic rumble

The murmur of MR is characterized by a holo-systolic murmur with a slightly split S2 and early A2

Mitral valve prolapse is characterized by a mid-systolic click followed by a murmur.

Aortic stenosis is described as a harsh systolic ejection murmur radiating to the carotids.

Aortic regurgitation is characterized by a diastolic decrescendo murmur.

The Valsalva maneuver will increase

the murmur of obstructive

cardiomyopathy.

The Valsalva maneuver will decrease the murmur of aortic stenosis.

The Valsalva maneuver will decrease

the murmur of mitral regurgitation

Squatting will decrease the murmur
of obstructive cardiomyopathy.

Squatting will increase the murmur of

aortic stenosis.

Squatting will increase the murmur of mitral regurgitation

Inspiration will increase the venous

return of blood to the heart.

Inspiration will increase the intensity

of right sided murmurs.

A wide split S2 can occur with mitral regurgitation, pulmonary stenosis, or in the setting of a right bundle branch block.

A paradoxical split S2 can occur because of aortic stenosis, tricuspid regurgitation, or in the setting of a left bundle branch block.

A fixed split S2 can occur because of an ASD or a VSD.

Right heart failure is characterized by peripheral edema and nocturia.

The physical exam findings of right heart failure are characterized by increased jugular venous distention, splenomegaly, and hepatomegaly.

Increased JVD is associated with biventricular failure, cardiac tamponade, constrictive pericarditis, Cor-pulmonale, and SVC syndrome.

Type of pain, onset of pain, precipitating factors, relieving factors, location, and duration of pain should be evaluated in patients with chest pain.

Non-sustained ventricular tachycardia is defined as three or more consecutive ventricular ectopic beats at a rate of >100 beats/min and lasting <30 seconds.

Monomorphic or polymorphic non-sustained ventricular tachycardia may be seen in up to 67% of patients during the first 12 hours after an acute myocardial infarction.

Episodes of sustained ventricular tachycardia during the first 48 hours following an acute MI have a hospital mortality of approximately 20%.

The serum potassium and magnesium should be monitored closely in patients who have had an acute myocardial infarction. Hypokalemia has been shown to increase the risk of developing ventricular tachycardia. The serum potassium level should be kept above 4.5 mEq/L and the serum magnesium above 2 mEq/L.

Cardiovascular related syncope is
caused by arrhythmias and
neurocardiogenic syncope

Patients with neurocardiogenic syncope develop a sudden and precipitous fall in both heart rate and blood pressure. In some patients, the blood pressure drops without a fall in heart rate. Neurocardiogenic syncope includes the vasovagal faint.

The typical symptoms of a vasovagal meditated syncopal episodes include lightheadedness, nausea, diaphoresis, salivation, pallor, tinnitus, and dimming of vision from vagal mediated hypotension and bradycardia.

Carotid sinus syncope develops secondary to vagal stimulation from the carotid sinus resulting in hypotension and/or bradycardia.

The most common complication of the PA catheter is arrhythmia.

Sustained ventricular tachycardia occur in approximately 3% with PA catheterizations

Rupture of the pulmonary artery occurs with right heart catheterization approximately 0.2% of the time.

PEA is continued electrical
rhythmicity of the heart in the
absence of effective mechanical
function.

Reversible causes of pulseless electrical activity include hypovolemia, hypoxia, cardiac tamponade, tension pneumothorax, hypothermia, massive pulmonary embolism, drug overdose, hyperkalemia, severe acidosis, and massive MI.

Pericardial tamponade should be considered in a patient presenting with pulseless electrical activity (PEA) and an elevated jugular venous pressure?

A large right sided x and y descent and the Kussmaul sign are most associated with constrictive pericarditis.

Equal diastolic readings will be identified in all 4 chambers in patients with constrictive pericarditis.

Kussmaul sign is the name given to increased jugular venous distension during inspiration.

Patients with pericarditis will describe an improvement in pain when they sit forward.

Ninety percent of non-constrictive

pericarditis are idiopathic.

The AST is elevated in 98% of
patients with acute MI's.

Celiac sprue, disorders of muscle metabolism, exercise, and muscle disease can all be associated with elevations in the AST.

Four causes of restrictive cardiomyopathy include endocardial fibro elastosis, endomyocardial fibrosis, amyloidosis and sarcoidosis.

The 4 components of the Eisenmenger's complex include right to left shunt, pulmonary hypertension, ventricular septal defect, and right ventricular hypertrophy.

About 25-30% of hypertrophic cardiomyopathy is autosomal dominant and 70% cryptogenic.

The four causes of dilated cardiomyopathy include ETOH toxicity, post viral myocarditis, peripartum cardiomyopathy, and chronic cocaine abuse.

Three causes of cardiomyopathies include dilated (congestive cardiomyopathy), hypertrophic cardiomyopathy, and restrictive/obliterative cardiomyopathy.

Four causes of acute pericarditis include infection, ischemic heart disease, chronic renal failure, and connective tissue diseases.

Infantile aortic stenosis occurs

proximal to insertion of ductus

arteriosus: Adult aortic stenosis

occurs distal to ductus arteriosus

Four findings of the tetralogy of Fallot include pulmonary stenosis, ventricular septal defect, right ventricular hypertrophy and overriding aorta.

Beta blockers often used in the setting of Marfan's syndrome to reduce the incidence of aortic aneurysms.

Five factors that can decrease cardiac compliance positive pressure ventilation, myocardial infarction, myocardial edema, ventricular hypertrophy, and pericardial tamponade.

The action of Norepinephrine is an agonist of Alpha 1, Alpha 2, B1, and increases ionotropy, increases chronotropy, and increases blood pressure.

Hypertrophic cardiomyopathy has an annual mortality rate of approximately 4%

EKG findings in the setting of atrial infarction include a depressed or elevated PR interval, atrial arrhythmias (atrial flutter and fibrillation), AV nodal rhythms, and depression or elevation of the PR interval.

Three weeks of anticoagulation is required if the atrial fibrillation is present for an unknown duration or greater than 48 hours.

Holiday heart is characterized by atrial fibrillation related to alcohol binges. These usually resolve after discontinuing alcohol for 48-72 hours.

Thrombosis in patients with atrial fibrillation has been associated with hypertension, diabetes, congestive heart failure, valvular heart disease, history of TIA, and age greater than 75.

The classic findings on auscultation of aortic regurgitation include S3 at the apex: Decrescendo blowing diastolic murmur at the left sternal border: Low-pitched apical diastolic rumble (Austin-Flint murmur): Early systolic apical ejection murmur

The physical exam finding suggestive of an inferior MI include hypotension, elevated jugular veins, and clear lungs.

The onset of CHF and a new systolic murmur 2 days after an acute non-Q-wave anterior lateral MI is suggestive of ventricular septal rupture and acute mitral insufficiency.

The 4 causes of ST elevation on an EKG include Acute transmural MI, ventricular aneurysm post MI, pericarditis, and Printzmal's angina.

Two characteristic EKG findings of a transmural myocardial infarction include Q waves of at least 0.04 seconds and inversion of T waves.

The 5 conditions are characterized by an increase in JVD include biventricular failure, cardiac tamponade, constrictive pericarditis, cor-Pulmonale, and SVC syndrome.

Right sided heart failure is associated with JVD, peripheral cyanosis, ascites, hepatic congestion, and hepatojugular reflux.

Left sided heart failure is associated with paradoxical splitting of S2 and S3, tachypnea, rales, and murmurs of MR, AS, and AR.

The two drugs most commonly associated with pericarditis include hydralazine and procainamide.

Three things can cause the PA waveform to dampen include wedged position, kink in the line, and clot at the end of the catheter.

Three medications that can aggravate carotid sinus hypersensitivity and lead to secondary syncope include beta blockers, methyldopa, and digoxin.

Two cardiac murmurs increase with the Valsalva maneuver include mitral valve prolapsed and hypertrophic obstructive cardiomyopathy

Four physical exam findings associated with mitral regurgitation include obliterated first heart sound, holosystolic murmur, widely split second heart sound, and at times a low pitched diastolic rumble.

Three causes of tricuspid stenosis include rheumatic heart disease, carcinoid syndrome, and atrial tumors.

Four symptoms that are commonly seen in constrictive pericarditis include peripheral edema, ascites, dyspnea, and fatigue.

The right sided murmurs (tricuspid regurgitation, pulmonary stenosis, and pulmonary regurgitation) are characterized by an increase of intensity of murmurs seen with inspiration (increase venous return).

Severe aortic stenosis is characterized by gradient of >50 mmhg and valve area of < 0.5 cm2.

Two conditions are associated with a bounding pulse include aortic regurgitation and A-V fistula.

The fourth heart sound is caused by the atria kick as blood is forced into a non-compliant ventricle. Four conditions in which the fourth heart sound could often be heard include ischemic heart disease, aortic stenosis, hypertension, and hypertrophic cardiomyopathy

Two causes of holosystolic murmurs include mitral regurgitation and ventricular septal defects.

Kussmaul sign seen is seen in pericardial tamponade and pericardial constriction.

: ECG findings of RV hypertrophy:
-R wave larger than S wave in V1
or V2 include R wave > 5mm in V1
or V2: R axis deviation: Persistent
rS pattern in V1-V6: Normal QRS
duration.

Contraindications to an exercise stress test: MI: Unstable angina: Acute myocarditis or pericarditis: Left main coronary disease: Severe aortic stenosis: Uncontrolled hypertension: Uncontrolled cardiac arrhythmia: Second or third degree heart block.

Right sided heart failure is associated with JVD, peripheral cyanosis, ascites, hepatic congestion, and hepatojugular reflux.

Left sided heart failure is associated with paradoxical splitting of S2 and S3, tachypnea, rales, and murmurs of MR and AS.

Mitral stenosis is characterized by a diastolic opening snap, loud S1, and a diastolic rumble.

Left heart failure is associated with dyspnea, orthopnea, and wheezing.

Patients with vasovagal mediated syncope develop lightheadedness, nausea, diaphoresis, salivation, pallor, tinnitus, and dimming of vision from vagally mediated hypotension and bradycardia.

A first degree AV block is present when there is >.20 second PR interval on the electrocardiogram.

Q waves of at least 0.04 seconds and inversion of T waves are two characteristic EKG findings of a transmural myocardial infarction.

The physical exam findings of an inferior MI include hypotension, elevated jugular veins, and clear lungs.

The murmur of MR is
characterized by a holosystolic
murmur with a slightly split S2 and
early A2.

Aortic stenosis is described as a harsh systolic ejection murmur radiating to the carotids.

Mitral valve prolapse is characterized by a mid-systolic click followed by a murmur.

Infantile aortic stenosis occurs proximal to insertion of ductus arteriosus.

Adult aortic stenosis occurs distal

to ductus arteriosus.

You would expect those patients who had successful cardiac reperfusion to reach higher peak levels of troponin at a faster rate when compared to those who were not successfully reperfused.

Carotid sinus syncope develops secondary to vagal stimulation from the carotid sinus resulting in hypotension and/or bradycardia.

Three common cardiomyopathies are dilated (congestive cardiomyopathy), hypertrophic cardiomyopathy, and restrictive/obliterative cardiomyopathy.

Blood aspirated from a pericardial effusion will not clot if is from the effusion.

A pacemaker is indicated in patients with Mobitz type I AV block only if the patient is symptomatic

A Mobitz II is indicated by a constant PR interval with a skip of the QRS.

T-wave inversion on an ECG can be either nonspecific, occur during ischemia, or occur after an MI.

Monomorphic or polymorphic non-sustained ventricular tachycardia may be seen in up to 67% of patients during the first 12 hours after an acute myocardial infarction.

ST elevation on an ECG is indicative
of transmural ischemia or coronary
artery spasm.

ST depression on an ECG is
consistent with subendocardial
ischemia.

Q waves on an ECG are indicative of a transmural infarction.

Atrial infarction is associated with depressed or elevated PR interval and atrial arrhythmias (A- flutter, A-fib, AV nodal rhythms).

EKG findings of ventricular tachycardia: -AV dissociation - Capture beats (normal conducted sinus beats interrupting a wide complex tachycardia) -Fusion beats (beats with qrs morphology intermediate between a normal narrow beat and a wide complex

Type of pain, onset of pain, precipitating factors, relieving factors, location, and duration of pain should be evaluated in patients presenting with chest discomfort.

Increased JVD is associated with biventricular failure, cardiac tamponade, and constrictive pericarditis, cor-pulmonale, and SVC syndrome.

Three conditions commonly associated with large A-waves are Tricuspid stenosis, Right ventricular hypertrophy, and pulmonary hypertension.

Approximately 3% of the time

sustained ventricular tachycardia

occur with PA catheterization.

Mitral valve prolapse and hypertrophic obstructive cardiomyopathy are two cardiac murmurs increase with the Valsalva maneuver.

Physical exam findings associated with mitral regurgitation:

-Obliterated first heart sound - holosystolic murmur

-widely split second heart sound

-at times a low pitched diastolic rumble.

Three causes of tricuspid stenosis:

-Rheumatic heart disease

-Carcinoid syndrome

-Atrial tumors

Symptoms commonly seen in constrictive pericarditis include peripheral edema, ascites, dyspnea, and fatigue.

Right sided murmurs (tricuspid regurgitation, pulmonary stenosis, and pulmonary regurgitation) are characterized by an increase of intensity of murmurs seen with inspiration (increase venous return).

Severe aortic stenosis is characterized by a valve gradient of >50 mmhg and a valve area of < 0.5 cm2.

Fixed splitting of S2 occurs when the interval between the closing of the aortic and pulmonic valves does not vary with inspiration and expiration. This can be seen in the setting of atrial septal defects and right ventricular dysfunction.

Kussmaul sign is seen in the setting of pericardial tamponade and pericardial constriction.

Non-sustained ventricular tachycardia is defined as three or more consecutive ventricular ectopic beats at a rate of >100 beats/min and lasting <30 seconds.

The fourth heart sound is caused by the atrial kick as blood is forced into a non-compliant ventricle.

The causes of 4th heart sound include Ischemic heart disease, aortic stenosis, hypertension, and hypertrophic cardiomyopathy.

Mitral regurgitation and ventricular septal defects are two causes of holosystolic murmurs.

Patients with neuro-cardiogenic syncope develop a sudden and precipitous fall in both heart rate and blood pressure. In some patients, the blood pressure drops without a fall in heart rate.

Arrhythmias and neurocardiogenic syncope
are the most common causes of
cardiovascular related syncope.

The serum potassium and magnesium should be monitored closely in post myocardial infarction patients.

Episodes of sustained ventricular tachycardia during the first 48 hours following an acute MI have a hospital mortality of approximately 20%.

Aortic regurgitation and A-V fistula are two conditions associated with a bounding pulse.

The cardiac catheterization findings in patients with constrictive pericarditis are characterized by equal diastolic readings will be identified in all 4 chambers.

Inspiration will increase the intensity

of right sided murmurs.

Ninety percent of non-constrictive

pericarditis are idiopathic.

Orthodromic reentrant tachycardia is the most common type of tachyarrhythmia seen in WPW.

Patients with pericarditis will describe an improvement in pain when they sit forward.

Ace inhibitors should not be given to

pregnant women.

Three atrial septal defects from high to low:

-Sinus venosus defect

-Ostium secundum defect

-Ostium primum defect

A paradoxical split S2 heart sound can occur in the setting of aortic stenosis, tricuspid regurgitation, or left bundle branch block.

The soft tissue densities consisting of aortic knob and a dilated descending aorta may form a '3 on CXR in patients with coarctation of the aorta. On barium swallow the esophagus may look like an 'E'

Hypokalemia can result in ECG changes, including ST depression, decreased amplitude of T-waves or inverted T-waves, increased amplitude of U waves, and prolongation of QT and PR interval.

Causes of narrow complex tachycardia include:

-Sinus tachycardia (less than 200 bpm with presence of p waves)

-Supraventricular tachycardia (>230 bpm with absence of p waves)

Large (cannon) A waves seen in the jugular venous pulse occur when the atria contract against a closed tricuspid valve. They are seen in the setting of A-V dissociation, ectopic atrial beats, and junctional or ventricular rhythms.

Patients with right ventricular MI's should avoid fluid restriction and diuretics because they depend on adequate preload to maintain LV function and adequate stroke volume.

Hypokalemia, hypocalcemia, hypomagnesaemia, and type 1A or 1C antiarrhythmic drugs (procainamide, quinidine, disopyramide, flecainide, and lidocaine) can be associated with QT prolongation.

ACE inhibitors have been associated with a decreased mortality following myocardial infarction, clinical improvement of CHF, and attenuation of left ventricular enlargement.

Side effects of ace inhibitors include cough, angioedema, laryngeoedema, neutropenia, metallic taste, and large drop in blood pressure after first dose.

Causes of decreased cardiac compliance include positive pressure ventilation, myocardial infarction, myocardial edema, ventricular hypertrophy, and pericardial tamponade.

A wide split S2 can occur with mitral regurgitation, pulmonary stenosis, or in the setting of a right bundle branch block.

Cardioversion restores sinus rhythm in 70 to 95 per cent of patients with atrial fibrillation. Sinus rhythm persists after 12 months in less than one-third to one-half the patients with cardioverted for chronic atrial fibrillation.

IV adenosine causes 2 second A-V heart block. In arrhythmias with reentrant circuits through the AV node (supraventricular), these rhythm will be terminated in patients with ventricular tachycardia they will not.

The exam findings of left heart failure

include S3 gallop and an S4 gallop.

Electrical alternans is the term that describes an alternating amplitude of the QRS complex in any or all leads associated with cardiac tamponade.

Beta blockers often used in the setting of Marfan's syndrome to reduce the incidence of aortic aneurysms.

Three weeks of anticoagulation is required prior to cardioversion if atrial fibrillation is present for an unknown duration or greater than 48 hours.

A fixed split S2 can occur because of

an ASD or a VSD.

The left ventricular end diastolic
pressure, left atrial pressure, and
left heart preload are all
representative of the pulmonary
capillary wedge pressure.

Aortic regurgitation is characterized by a diastolic decrescendo murmur.

EKG findings in the setting of atrial infarction include a depressed or elevated PR interval, atrial arrhythmias (atrial flutter and fibrillation), AV nodal rhythms, and depression or elevation of the PR interval.

Pericardial tamponade should be considered in a patient presenting with pulseless electrical activity (PEA) and an elevated jugular venous pressure.

The reversible causes of pulseless electrical activity include hypovolemia, hypoxia, cardiac tamponade, tension pneumothorax, hypothermia, massive pulmonary embolism, drug overdose, hyperkalemia, severe acidosis, and massive MI.

PEA is continued electrical rhythmicity of the heart in the absence of effective mechanical function.

Squatting will increase the murmur of

mitral regurgitation.

Inspiration will increase the venous

return of blood to the heart.

Fluid overload, pulmonary embolus, myocardial infarction, and pain are commonly associated with post-operative atrial fibrillation.

Second degree heart block is characterized by intermittent AV conduction blocks with failure to propagate the impulse to the ventricle.

Mobitz II is usually associated with a bundle branch block. The PR intervals are constant before and after the dropped P wave.

Thrombosis in the setting of atrial fibrillation has been associated with hypertension, diabetes, congestive heart failure, valvular heart disease, history of TIA, and age greater than 75.

Digitalis toxicity, vomiting, pain, straining to void, and gagging can all increase the vagal tone and result in transient second degree heart block.

Squatting will increase the murmur of aortic stenosis.

Squatting will decrease the murmur of obstructive cardiomyopathy.

Digitalis increases the refractory period of the AV node and increases the excitability and automaticity in the Perkinge's fibers.

Heart block or ventricular arrhythmias can develop in the setting of digitalis toxicity.

The Valsalva maneuver will decrease

the murmur of aortic stenosis.

The Valsalva maneuver will increase the murmur of obstructive cardiomyopathy.

Hyperkalemia, acute renal failure, chronic cough, and angioedema are side effects of ACE inhibitors.

The structural and functional benefits of ACE inhibitors used in the setting of post MI or early left ventricular dysfunction include decreased transmural wall stress, decreased compensatory dilatation and increased coronary flow distribution.

The hemodynamic benefits of ACE inhibitors used in the setting of post MI or early left ventricular dysfunction include decreased vascular resistance, decreased ionotropic stimulation, and decreased chronotropic stimulation.

Two EKG findings typical of

ventricular tachycardia:

-AV dissociation

-Fusion beats

Fixed splitting of S2 occurs when the interval between the closing of the aortic and pulmonic valves does not vary with inspiration and expiration. This can be seen in the setting of atrial septal defects and right ventricular dysfunction.

Standing results in increased left ventricular outflow obstruction and an increase in murmur intensity in IHSS.

EKG evolution after MI include:

-Tall T waves are seen in the first 1-2 hours (T wave inversion usually after ST segment elevation has occurred)

-ST elevation in leads facing the infarcted myocardium and depression occurs in opposite leads

-Q waves develop in hours to days.

The QT interval is determined by the heart rate, and because the rate can vary, we calculate the corrected QT (QTc): QTc = Q-T (seconds) / square root of R-R interval (seconds): Normal is 0.32-0.44 seconds.

Differential diagnosis of congestive heart failure in a hypertensive patient:

Coronary artery disease

Diastolic dysfunction

Dilated cardiomyopathy (idiopathic vs. Alcoholic)

Valvular heart disease (MR, AS, AI)

Restrictive heart disease (Amyloid)

Hypertrophic cardiomyopathy

The hemodynamic benefits of ACE inhibitors used in the setting of post MI or early left ventricular dysfunction:

Decrease vascular resistance

Decrease ionotropic stimulation

Decrease chronotropic stimulation

The structural and functional benefits of ACE inhibitors used in the setting of post MI or early left ventricular dysfunction:

Decrease transmural wall stress

Decrease compensatory dilatation

Increase coronary flow distribution

The 4 etiologies of ST elevation on an EKG:

Acute transmural MI

Ventricular aneurysm post MI

Pericarditis

Printzmal's angina

The characteristic EKG findings of a transmural MI:

-Q waves of at least 0.04 seconds

-Inversion of T waves

Men are more likely to develop aortic
aneurysms 10:1 over women.

The most common symptom of an aortic dissection is intrascapular back pain

Approximately 2/3 of post-operative MI's likely occur on post-op day 2-5.

Two reasons for new onset of CHF and a new systolic murmur 2 days after an acute non-Q wave anterolateral MI:

Ventricular septal rupture

Acute mitral insufficiency

Fusion beats on an EKG in ventricular tachycardia occurs when an atrial impulse initiates ventricular depolarization simultaneously with onset of an ectopic ventricular beat.

The brain, heart, and adrenal glands preferentially receive blood flow during periods of mild asphyxia.

Abnormal wide splitting of S2 can be seen in:

Right ventricular overload

Right ventricular conduction delay

Prolonged right ventricular emptying

Three types of cardiovascular shock:

Hypovolemic

Cardiogenic

Distributive

Smoking is the strongest risk factor for claudication

Dobutamine is a beta 1 and beta 2 agonist which results in increased ionotropy and increased chronotropy.

Digitalis increases the refractory period of the AV node and increases the excitability and automaticity in the Perkinge's fibers leading to heart block or ventricular arrhythmias

Familial hypercholesterolemia is an autosomal dominant disease is associated with a mutant LDL receptor that is characterized by premature atherosclerosis and tendon xanthomas

Four effects of hypokalemia on the
electrocardiogram:

-ST depression

-Decreased amplitude of T-waves or
inverted T-waves

-Increased amplitude of U waves

-Prolongation of QT and PR interval

3 classes of drugs are associated with tachyarrhythmics and secondary syncope:

-Antiarrhythmic

-Tricyclic antidepressants

-Phenothiazine

The most common right heart valvular disorder is tricuspid regurgitation.

Infectious endocarditis is the most

common cause of acute aortic

insufficiency.

The symptoms of aortic stenosis generally begin to occur when the valve area is <1.0 cm2.

The Valsalva increases intra-thoracic pressure, thus inhibiting venous return to the right heart.

Approximately 250 ml of pericardial effusion is needed before it can be seen on a chest x-ray.

Ebstein's anomaly is characterized by the inferior displacement of the tricuspid valve ring into the ventricular cavity.

William's syndrome is the genetic syndrome characterized by supra-valvular aortic stenosis, elfin facies, mental retardation, and hypercalcemia.

Hypertrophic cardiomyopathy is associated with a trifid point of maximal impulse.

The etiology of the first heart sound
is mitral valve closure followed closely
by tricuspid closure.

Mitral stenosis is associated with a loud first heart sound with a short PR interval

Coronary artery disease is the most common cause of CHF.

Acute myocardial infarction is the most common cause of cardiogenic shock.

IV verapamil contraindicated in the setting of digitalis toxicity because digoxin and verapamil both inhibit the AV node.

Hypokalemia, hypocalcemia, hypomagnesaemia, and type 1A or 1C antiarrhythmic drugs (procainamide, quinidine, disopyramide, flecainide, and lidocaine) can be associated with QT prolongation.

The findings on a right sided ECG of a right sided MI include greater than 1mm of ST elevation in V3R and V4R

Pulsus paradoxus is the disappearance of the pulse during inspiration despite persistence of a heartbeat.

Patients with a right ventricular MI should avoid fluid restriction and diuretics because they depend on adequate preload to maintain LV function and adequate stroke volume.

Aortic sclerosis is the most common cause of a systolic ejection murmur at the right upper sternal border.

The split second heart sound is caused by the time interval between the closing of the aortic and pulmonic valves.

Non transmural MI is indicated by depressed ST segments or symmetric T-wave inversions on an EKG

Beck's triad is characterized by an elevated JVD, distant heart sounds, and low blood pressure

ACE inhibitors have been associated with a decreased mortality following myocardial infarction, clinical improvement of CHF, and attenuation of left ventricular enlargement.

Magnesium sulfate is used to safely and effectively convert patients with torsade de pointes due to acquired QT prolongation

Patients with hypertrophic cardiomyopathy can present with a systolic murmur which is reduced in intensity when the patient squats.

NSAIDS decrease the
antihypertensive effects of ACE
inhibitors.

The annual risk of stroke in a patient with atrial fibrillation who is less than 60 without hypertension, history of embolism, diabetes, or depressed ejection fraction is about 0.5%-1%/year.

Atrioventricular nodal reentrant tachycardia is the most common form of PSVT and accounts for 50-60% of PSVT

Orthodromic reentrant tachycardia is the most common type of tachyarrhythmia seen in WPW. The electrical impulse is conducted through the AV node and the His-Purkinje system in the normal antegrade direction to activate the ventricular myocardium and returns to the atria via the accessory connection.

ACE-inhibitor related cough is caused
an increase in bradykinin.

Gemfibrozil is a fibric acid derivative that decreases VLDL-TG synthesis and increases VLDL-TG clearance.

Magnesium deficiency has been associated with ventricular and supraventricular dysrhythmias.

Cyanosis of mucous membranes is diagnostic of a right to left cardiac shunt

Ejection murmurs are associated with aortic and pulmonary valve stenosis.

Mitral valve prolapsed is associated with a late systolic murmur.

The ductus arteriosus connects the pulmonary artery with the descending aorta.

Carotid and femoral pulses indicate a systolic blood pressure of at least 60 mmhg.

Fluid overload, pulmonary embolus, myocardial infarction, and pain are commonly associated with post-operative atrial fibrillation.

The second heart sound is caused by aortic closure followed by pulmonic closure.

Hypertension increases the intensity of the second heart sound.

Second degree heart block is characterized by intermittent AV conduction blocks with failure to propagate the impulse to the ventricle

Digitalis toxicity, vomiting, pain, straining to void, and gagging can all increase the vagal tone and result in transient second degree heart block.

Aortic stenosis is characterized by a loud systolic murmur heard best at the base and transmitted to the carotids.

Electrical alternans is a variably alternating amplitude of the QRS complex in any or all leads commonly associated with cardiac tamponade.

Cor pulmonale is right ventricle enlargement secondary to pulmonary hypertension.

Pulmonary embolus is the most common cause of acute cor pulmonale.

It takes approximately 3-6 hours for cardiac troponins to appear in the blood after a myocardial infarction.

It takes approximately 10-24 hours for cardiac troponins to reach peak levels after a myocardial infarction.

It takes approximately 0.5-2 hours for myoglobin to appear in the blood after a myocardial infarction.

It takes approximately 3-8 hours for CPK-MB to appear in the blood after a myocardial infarction.

Approximately 85% of patients having an MI will show evidence on the EKG.

The most common cause of aortic
stenosis is congenital bicuspid aortic
valve.

Idiopathic hypertrophic sub aortic stenosis is most commonly inherited autosomal dominant.

Pericardial effusion is characteristic of a "water bottle" appearance on the chest radiograph.

Pulsus paradoxus is the physical exam finding most consistent with pericardial tamponade

Greater than 200 ml of fluid is needed in the pericardial sac is needed for the development of acute pericardial tamponade.

Persistence of ostium secundum is the most common atrial septal defect, accounting for approximately 80% of patients.

Cardiac tamponade can be characterized by low voltage, electrical alternans, and PR depression on an ECG

The half-life of digoxin is 30-50 hours and the half-life of digitoxin is 5-8 days.

It takes approximately 6-10 days take
for total CPK levels in the blood to
return to normal after a myocardial
infarction.

Celiac sprue, disorders of muscle metabolism, exercise, and muscle disease can all be associated with elevations in the AST

You would expect those patients who were successfully reperfused to reach higher peak levels of troponin at a faster rate when compared to those who were not successfully reperfused.

This concludes Cardiology: Fast Focus Study Guide

Search Amazon Kindle books to find other study guides written by

JT Thomas, MD

Internal Medicine Study Guide

Medical Oncology Study Guide

Multiple Myeloma Study Guide

Differential Diagnosis Study Guide

Rheumatology Study Guide